# Keto Slow Cooker Made Easy

## 50 Delicious Low Carb Recipes To Help You Lose Weight Fast!

### Jen Smith

# Copyright Notice

All content is solely owned by the publisher and author of this book. No part of this book may be reproduced in any form by any electronic or mechanical means (including photocopying, recording, or information storage, and retrieval) without permission in writing from the publisher.

# Medical Disclaimer

All information, ideas and guidelines mentioned in this eBook are for informational purposes only. This publication cannot be used as a substitute for professional medical advice. The nutrition or fitness guidelines mentioned in this book do not take individual circumstances into consideration so they may not be appropriate in your case.

**Please consult with your doctor before following any advice in this book.**

No information in this book is intended to be medical diagnoses or advice. This book should never be used as medical advice or used in place of a visit to a medical professional. Always seek the advice of your physician or other qualified health provider prior to starting any new diet or treatment and with any questions you may have regarding a medical condition. If you have or suspect that you have a medical problem, promptly contact your health care provider.

This book is not intended to replace medical or health advice from a licensed physician. None of the information on this book should be considered medical diagnosis or treatment.

The author and publisher have taken utmost care to confirm the accuracy of the content; however, all readers are encouraged to follow the information at their own risk. The author and publisher cannot be held responsible for any personal or commercial damage that results from misinterpretation of information, negligence or otherwise. Always consult your healthcare professional if you have questions regarding specific medical conditions, or before starting a new diet.

If you are following the keto diet for any medical reason you should consult a qualified medical professional beforehand. Using this book is not a substitute for reading ingredient statements.

# Table of Contents

Introduction ............................................................................... 1
Chapter 1: Ketogenic Breakfast Recipes ............................. 3
    Ketogenic Breakfast Casserole ............................................ 3
    Butternut Squash Breakfast Casserole .............................. 4
    Egg and Bacon Breakfast Casserole ................................... 5
    Chili Pepper and Spinach Egg Casserole ........................... 6
    Kickin' Kale Frittata ............................................................... 7
Chapter 2: Appetizer Ketogenic Recipes ............................. 8
    Spicy Blue Cheese Dip ........................................................... 8
    Broccoli Cheddar Ketogenic Dip ......................................... 9
    Spinach and Artichoke Ketogenic Dip ............................. 10
    Party People Low-Carb Pizza Dip ..................................... 11
    Low-Carb Ketogenic Reuben Sandwich Dip ................... 12
    Crabmeat Northeastern Dip ............................................... 13
    Ketogenic Appetizer Honey Wings ................................... 14
Chapter 3: Chicken Ketogenic Recipes ............................. 15
    Slow Cooker Mandarin Chicken ........................................ 15
    Keto Chicken and Bacon Chili Soup ................................. 16
    Zucchini Pad Thai ................................................................. 17
    Buffalo-Inspired Chicken Slow Cooker Recipe ................ 18
    Chicken and Bacon Vegetable Chowder ........................... 19
    Gluten-Free Ketogenic Chicken Soup .............................. 20
    Lemon and Green Olive Chicken ....................................... 21
    Southern-Jerk Slow-Cooked Chicken ............................... 22
    Mediterranean Life Stuffed Chicken ................................ 23
    Low-Carb Ketogenic Cocoa Chicken Mole ....................... 24

Roasted Chicken and Faux Ketogenic Gravy ....................... 25
Chicken-Based Slow Cooker Pizza ........................................ 26

Chapter 4: Beef Ketogenic Recipes ............................................ 27
Irish Slow Cooker Corned Beef and Cabbage ..................... 27
Slow Cooker Beef-Based Pizza ............................................. 28
Faux Italian Meatball Soup .................................................. 29
BBQ-Based Pot Roast ........................................................... 30
Super Ketogenic Vegetable and Beef Chili ......................... 31
Faux Cheese Beef-Based Lasagna ....................................... 32
Ketogenic Chipotle Beef ....................................................... 34

Chapter 5: Pork Ketogenic Recipes ........................................... 35
Pork-Based Chili Recipe ....................................................... 35
Faux Split Pea and Ham Soup ............................................. 36
Apple Flavored Pork Tenderloin ......................................... 37
Mexican Style Pork Carnitas ............................................... 38
Classic Ketogenic Pulled Pork ............................................. 39
Pork-Stuffed Green Peppers ................................................ 40
Pork Sausage with Collared Greens ................................... 41
Super Peppered Pork Stew .................................................. 42

Chapter 6: Lamb Ketogenic Recipes ......................................... 43
Low-Carb Ketogenic Lamb with Tarragon ........................ 43
Slow Cooked Lamb Chops ................................................... 44
Crock Pot Braised Lamb ...................................................... 45
Moroccan-Based Lamb Stew Recipe .................................. 46
Down on the Farm Lamb Stew ........................................... 47

Chapter 7: Seafood Ketogenic Recipes ..................................... 48
Herbed and Poached Slow Cooked Salmon ....................... 48

Savory Shrimp Stew ............................................................. 49
Ketogenic Jambalaya ........................................................... 50
Chapter 8: Ketogenic Dessert Recipes ................................... 51
Autumnal Pumpkin Pie Cake ............................................. 52
Super Low-Carb Chocolate Fudge ...................................... 53
Conclusion ............................................................................. 54

# Introduction

The ketogenic diet is an essential tool utilized by fitness instructors, bodybuilders, people looking to lose weight, and even people who are riddled with diseases like Alzheimer's and cancer. The diet is generally low-carbohydrate and high-fat. It fuels you with protein and helps your body look to already-stored body fat for extra energy. When your body utilizes your stored ketones in your body, you aren't using glucose anymore; instead, you're using ketones. Ketones in your blood stream don't push your insulin levels too high, allowing you to lose fat and look your best.

**Some Helpful Benefits of the Ketogenic Diet:**

Look to the following to better understand where your body will be in a few short weeks with the ketogenic diet.

1. Lower blood sugar will decrease your risk of disease.

Studies show that people who have high blood pressure are more at risk for various cancers and Alzheimer's. When your body is ripe with ketones instead of glucose, your risks go down.

2. Your levels of bad cholesterol and bad body fat will go down immediately.

Your body, ripe with ketones, will look first toward body fat and bad cholesterol for energy rather than your muscle. Therefore, your body will lean up, tone up, and deliver you with a healthy frame for exercise and feeling great.

3. Your hunger levels will decrease rapidly, leaving you without cravings.

If you struggle with food cravings, the ketogenic diet is perfect for you. This is because protein and fat work to keep you satiated.

In order to begin your ketogenic diet, it's essential that you immediately limit your carbohydrate intake. The ketogenic diet looks to have you eat only 5% carbohydrates—from vegetables and fruits, 30% protein, and 65% fat. Remember that it will take you about thirty days to completely assimilate into the diet plan.

In order to understand if you're in ketosis, you need to buy Keto Sticks from your local drug store. You simply pee on the Keto Sticks to discover how many ketones or fat energy particles exist in your body. This means that when you pee fat from your system, you are consistently losing weight. Pretty awesome, no?

Look to the following 50 Slow Cooker Ketogenic recipes to lose weight, start burning fat on the daily, and cut down on your sugar and carbohydrate cravings immediately. Note that the slow cooker recipes are essential for you if you're trying to lose weight on a time constraint. Finally: an immediate answer for after-work, after school, or late night healthy meals!

# Chapter 1: Ketogenic Breakfast Recipes

## Ketogenic Breakfast Casserole

This sausage-based green pepper and spinach egg casserole is literally perfect for a big group of hungry morning people.

**Ingredients:**

- 15 ounces ground sausage
- 12 eggs
- 1 diced onion
- 1 diced green pepper
- 3 cups spinach
- 1 cup heavy cream
- 10 ounces shredded cheddar cheese
- 1 tsp. onion powder
- 1 tsp. garlic powder

**Directions:**

Begin by stirring all the ingredients together in the slow cooker, making sure to whip up the eggs. Allow the casserole to cook on LOW for seven hours. Slice and enjoy!

# Butternut Squash Breakfast Casserole

This soft-squash casserole is humming with rich flavor.

## Ingredients:

- 1 1/3 cup coconut milk
- 1 1/3 pound ground sausage
- 1 diced onion
- 12 eggs
- 1 diced butternut squash
- ½ tbsp. ghee

## Directions:

Begin by bringing every ingredient together in the slow cooker. Stir for a moment, place the lid on the slow cooker, and cook on LOW for four hours. Slice it up, and enjoy!

# Egg and Bacon Breakfast Casserole

This bacon-based egg casserole is super-easy for a busy college student or a person who has trouble in the kitchen.

## Ingredients:

- ¾ pounds ground turkey sausage
- ¾ cup bacon
- 8 eggs
- 1 diced onion
- ¼ cubed sweet potato
- 2 minced garlic cloves

## Directions:

Bring the above ingredients together in a slow cooker and cook them together on LOW for eight hours. Enjoy!

# Chili Pepper and Spinach Egg Casserole

Spicy chili peppers brighten this egg casserole on a rainy day.

## Ingredients:

- 8 eggs
- 3 diced tomatoes
- 1 diced onion
- 8 strips of bacon
- 3 cups spinach
- 2 chopped chilies
- 1 tbsp. coconut oil
- salt and pepper to taste

## Directions:

Bring all the ingredients together in the slow cooker, making sure to completely whisk the eggs. Allow the ingredients to cook on LOW for eight hours, and serve warm. Enjoy!

# Kickin' Kale Frittata

All the nutrition of kale is met with the fatty flavor of feta and eggs.

## Ingredients:

- 2 tbsp. olive oil
- 6 ounces kale
- 7 ounces diced roasted red peppers
- 1/3 cup diced onion
- 6 ounces diced Feta
- 9 eggs
- 1 tsp. basil
- salt and pepper to taste

## Directions:

Bring the above ingredients together in a slow cooker, making sure to beat together the eggs. Cook the frittata on LOW for three hours. The cheese should be melted. Enjoy!

# Chapter 2:
# Appetizer Ketogenic Recipes

## Spicy Blue Cheese Dip

This ketogenic buffalo blue cheese dip is an essential low-carb, ketogenic appetizer.

**Ingredients:**

- 10 ounces cream cheese
- 1 cup diced chicken breasts
- ½ cup Buffalo sauce
- 1 diced celery stalk
- 1 minced jalapeno chili pepper
- 2 tbsp. blue cheese salad dressing

**Directions:**

Begin by bringing the above ingredients together in a slow cooker. Stir well, and place the lid on the slow cooker. Allow the mixture to cook on LOW for four hours. After four hours, stir well, and serve with vegetables. Enjoy!

# Broccoli Cheddar Ketogenic Dip

This salsa and bacon-based broccoli cheddar dip is super flavorful and perfect with some of the later ketogenic chili recipes.

## Ingredients:

- 10 ounces cream cheese
- 2 cups diced broccoli
- 8 ounces shredded cheddar cheese
- 4 tsp. bacon bits
- 4 tbsp. salsa

## Directions:

Bring all the above ingredients together in the slow cooker, and stir well. Next, place the lid on the slow cooker, and allow it to cook on LOW for five hours. Stir well, and enjoy!

# Spinach and Artichoke Ketogenic Dip

This ketogenic take on the classic spinach and artichoke dip will treat your taste buds.

## Ingredients:

- 5 minced garlic cloves
- 1 ½ cup shredded Mozzarella
- 10 ounces frozen spinach
- 10 ounces pasta sauce
- 14 ounces artichoke hearts
- ½ cup grated Parmesan cheese
- 8 ounces cream cheese

## Directions:

Begin by stirring all of the above ingredients together in the slow cooker. Place the lid on the slow cooker, and allow it to cook for four hours on LOW. Stir well, and enjoy!

# Party People Low-Carb Pizza Dip

Parmesan, Mozzarella, and pizza sauce spin together in this awesome pizza dip.

## Ingredients:

- 10 ounces cream cheese
- 1 ¼ cup Parmesan cheese
- ¼ tsp. parsley
- ½ tsp. oregano
- 1 ¼ cup pizza sauce
- ½ diced green pepper
- 3 ounces diced pepperoni
- 1 tbsp. diced olives
- ¾ cup Mozzarella cheese

## Directions:

Begin by mixing together all the ingredients in a slow cooker. Cook the ingredients on LOW for three hours. Stir well, and serve warm. Enjoy!

# Low-Carb Ketogenic Reuben Sandwich Dip

A ketogenic reuben-based dip is all your snack time needs.

## Ingredients:

- 10 ounces shredded corned beef
- 1/3 cup mayonnaise
- 15 ounces squeezed dry sauerkraut
- 1/3 cup Thousand Island dressing
- 15 ounces shredded Swiss cheese

## Directions:

Bring the above ingredients together into a slow cooker, and stir well. Next, place the lid on the slow cooker and allow the mixture to cook on LOW for six hours. Enjoy warm!

## Crabmeat Northeastern Dip

Creamy crab dip for your next New Years Eve celebration!

### Ingredients:

- 2 cups shredded Parmesan cheese
- 8 ounces canned crabmeat
- 8 ounces cream cheese
- ¾ cup sour cream
- 5 minced garlic cloves
- 1 ¼ cup mayonnaise

### Directions:

Begin by bringing all of the above ingredients together into your slow cooker. Stir well, and place the lid on the slow cooker. Next, cook the ingredients on LOW for four hours. Stir well, and then place the lid on the slow cooker. Escalate the het to HIGH and cook for another thirty minutes before serving. Enjoy!

# Ketogenic Appetizer Honey Wings

These simplistic honey and garlic-based chicken wings brighten any mood: even when your team is losing.

## Ingredients:

- 3 pounds chicken wings
- 1 cup raw honey
- 2 tbsp. minced garlic
- 1 ½ tbsp. olive oil
- salt and pepper

## Directions:

1. Bring the wings into the slow cooker.
2. To the side, mix together all the other ingredients. Pour this mixture over the wings and stir well.
3. Cook the wings on LOW for seven hours, and enjoy warm!

# Chapter 3:
# Chicken Ketogenic Recipes

## Slow Cooker Mandarin Chicken

This garlic and ginger-based chicken is pulsing with Asian-inspired flavor.

**Ingredients:**

- 5 chicken thighs
- 1 ½ tbsp. Chinese five spice powder
- 1 tsp. salt
- 1 ¼ cup mandarin oranges
- 1 tsp. red chilies
- 1 ½ tbsp. ginger
- 3 tbsp. fish sauce
- ½ tsp. sesame oil
- 1 tbsp. lime juice

**Directions:**

Begin by rubbing the five spices powder over the chicken. Place the chicken in the slow cooker along with the rest of the ingredients, and stir well. Cook this mixture on LOW for six hours. Next, remove the chicken from the slow cooker and place it on a plate. Blend the other goop from the slow cooker in a blender until completely smooth, and pour this mixture over the chicken. Enjoy.

# Keto Chicken and Bacon Chili Soup

This chili is perfect for a cold winter day; it's revving with lemon and thyme flavor.

**Ingredients:**

- 3 tbsp. butter
- 1 diced green pepper
- 1 diced onion
- 2 tbsp. thyme
- 10 slices bacon
- 7 boneless chicken thighs
- 1 tbsp. coconut flour
- ½ tbsp. garlic
- 1 cup chicken stock
- 4 tbsp. lemon juice
- 1/3 cup coconut milk
- 4 tbsp. tomato paste

**Directions:**

Bring everything together into the slow cooker, stir several times, and allow it to cook on LOW for six hours. Enjoy warm.

# Zucchini Pad Thai

This zucchini-based pad Thai contains all the flavor of your favorite dish—without the carbs.

**Ingredients:**

- 2 ½ pounds chicken breasts
- 1 carrot
- 2 zucchini
- 1 up coconut milk
- 2 diced onions
- 2 tbsp. sunbutter
- 1 cup chicken stock
- 1 tbsp. coconut aminos
- 2 diced garlic cloves
- 2 tsp. ginger
- 3 tsp. Fish sauce
- salt and pepper to taste

**Directions:**

Begin by salting and peppering and spicing up the chicken. Next, make noodles with the zucchini and slice and dice the other vegetables. Bring everything together in the slow cooker, and cook the pad Thai for four hours on LOW. Serve warm, without the created liquid. Slice and dice the meat, as well, and enjoy.

# Buffalo-Inspired Chicken Slow Cooker Recipe

Southwest buffalo flavor is electric in this chicken recipe.

## Ingredients:

- 5 chicken breasts
- 1 packet of ranch
- ½ cup Frank's red hot sauce
- 4 tbsp. butter

## Directions:

Bring all the ingredients together in the slow cooker and stir well. Cover the chicken and allow it to cook for six hours on LOW. Next, shred the chicken and serve warm. Enjoy.

# Chicken and Bacon Vegetable Chowder

This smooth and creamy chowder takes you back to the east coast waves.

**Ingredients:**

- 5 minced garlic cloves
- 1 ½ pound skinless and boneless chicken breasts
- 1 diced shallot
- 5 ounces sliced mushrooms
- 3 diced celery stalks
- 5 tbsp. butter
- 8 ounces cream cheese
- 1 ½ cup heavy cream
- 1 tsp. garlic powder
- salt and pepper to taste

**Directions:**

Bring all the above ingredients together, stir, and allow them to cook together on LOW for eight hours. Slice and tear up the chicken, and enjoy.

# Gluten-Free Ketogenic Chicken Soup

This gluten-free ketogenic chicken soup will get your metabolism revving immediately.

**Ingredients:**

- 1 diced yellow pepper
- 1 diced orange pepper
- 1 diced onion
- 2 pounds chicken breast
- 1 can diced tomatoes
- 32 ounces gluten-free chicken stock
- 7 ounces sliced mushrooms
- 4 tbsp. taco seasoning
- 5 minced garlic cloves
- 1 tbsp. salt

**Directions:**

Begin by bringing all the ingredients together in the slow cooker. Cook the ingredients for six hours on LOW. Next, shred the chicken and serve the soup warm. Enjoy!

# Lemon and Green Olive Chicken

This lemon-based chicken is vibrant with ingredients like fennel, green olives, and oregano.

**Ingredients:**

- 10 boneless chicken breasts
- 15 green olives
- 3 diced carrots
- 1 diced onion
- 1 diced fennel
- 3 diced celery stalks
- 1 tsp. oregano
- 3 tbsp. lemon juice
- 1/8 flour
- 1 cup chicken broth
- salt and pepper to taste

**Directions:**

Begin by bringing all the above ingredients together into the slow cooker. Cook the chicken on LOW for six hours. Afterwards, stir well and allow the mixture to thicken. Cook the chicken for an additional twenty minutes. Next, serve the chicken and the vegetables warm—without the juices—and enjoy!

# Southern-Jerk Slow-Cooked Chicken

This garlic and cardamom-slathered jerk chicken is an essential recipe in your keto toolkit.

## Ingredients:

- 4 ½ pounds chicken breasts
- 8 diced scallions
- 1 inch diced ginger
- 1/3 cup vegetable oil
- 1 tbsp. thyme
- 4 minced garlic cloves
- 1 tsp. salt
- 1 tsp. cardamom
- 3 tbsp. molasses

## Directions:

Bring the ingredients—except for the chicken—together in a food processor and process them well to create a sauce. Bring these ingredients and the chicken together in the slow cooker, and cook the chicken for five hours on LOW. Enjoy warm with extra sauce overtop.

# Mediterranean Life Stuffed Chicken

These vibrant Mediterranean chickens breasts are revving with high fats, high protein, and low carbohydrate value.

**Ingredients:**

- 6 chicken breasts
- 1/3 cup sliced olive
- 4 cups chopped spinach
- 3 diced red peppers
- 5 ounces feta cheese
- 1 ½ cup diced artichoke hearts
- 2 cups chicken broth
- 1 minced garlic clove
- salt and pepper

**Directions:**

1. Begin by mixing together the red peppers, the feta, the olives, the artichoke hearts, the spinach, and the garlic in a small bowl.
2. Next, slice open the chicken on the side and stuff the chicken with the created mixture. Place the chicken in the slow cooker and pour over the chicken broth.
3. Next, cook the chicken on LOW for four and a half hours. Enjoy warm!

# Low-Carb Ketogenic Cocoa Chicken Mole

This cocoa chicken mole will fuel your kitchen with delicious smells and bring your body into ketogenic, weight loss revving power.

**Ingredients:**

- 1 ¾ pounds chicken breasts
- 1 diced onion
- 2 ½ tbsp. ghee
- 5 minced garlic cloves
- 6 diced chili peppers
- 1/3 cup almond butter
- 3 ounces dark chocolate
- 7 diced tomatoes
- ½ tsp. cinnamon
- 1 tsp. cumin

**Directions:**

1. Brown the chicken first in the skillet with the ghee.
2. Next, place the chicken in the slow cooker and piece it up with a knife. Add the rest of the ingredients, and cook the mole on LOW for six hours. Tear the chicken apart, and enjoy warm.

# Roasted Chicken and Faux Ketogenic Gravy

This roasted chicken is complete with this delicious, thick, super ketogenic gravy that's perfect for your holiday meals!

**Ingredients:**

- 4 ½ pounds of chicken
- 3 diced onions
- 3 tbsp. ghee
- 1 tsp. tomato paste
- 7 minced garlic cloves
- 1/3 cup chicken stock
- 1 tsp. basil
- 1/3 cup white wine
- salt and pepper to taste

**Directions:**

1. Begin by bringing all the above ingredients together in the slow cooker. Allow the chicken to cook on LOW for five hours.
2. Next, remove the chicken and allow it to sit to the side. Pour the remaining ingredients together in a blender and blend them together to form the awesome gravy. Enjoy!

# Chicken-Based Slow Cooker Pizza

Crock pot chicken with pepperoni provides electric flavor for your next movie night.

## Ingredients:

- 2 ½ cups no-sugar pizza sauce
- 5 diced boneless chicken breasts
- 1 cup shredded Mozzarella cheese
- 18 slices pepperoni

## Directions:

Pour the sauce into the bottom of the slow cooker. Add the chicken and add the pepperoni overtop. Cook the pizza on LOW for four hours. Next, add the cheese to the top and place the lid back on the slow cooker. Allow it to cook for ten more minutes, and enjoy!

# Chapter 4: Beef Ketogenic Recipes

## Irish Slow Cooker Corned Beef and Cabbage

Irish life is yours with this slow cooker corned beef and cabbage recipe.

**Ingredients:**

- 1 diced onion
- 5 diced carrots
- 1 diced celery stalk
- 1 tsp. mustard
- 5 cups water
- 1 tsp. coriander
- salt and pepper
- ½ tsp. thyme
- ½ tsp. marjoram
- 6 pounds corned beef
- 1 head of cabbage

**Directions:**

1. Begin by bringing all the spices onto the beef and rubbing it well. Next, bring all the ingredients into the slow cooker, making sure to quarter the cabbage.
2. Next, cook the ingredients on LOW for seven hours, and enjoy warm.

# Slow Cooker Beef-Based Pizza

Mozzarella cheese melts evenly across this essential party pizza.

## Ingredients:

- 1 pound cooked ground beef
- 4 cups mozzarella cheese
- 1 pound Italian sausage
- 1 jar pizza sauce
- 4 cups spinach
- 15 slices of pepperoni

## Directions:

Begin by cooking up the sausage and the beef in a skillet for about five minutes. Next, assemble the pizza by pouring all of the burger and the sausage in the bottom of the slow cooker. Add half of the pizza sauce overtop followed by half of the spinach. Then, add half of the pepperoni and half of the mozzarella over these ingredients. Repeat the layers, and then allow the pizza to cook on LOW for six hours. Enjoy!

# Faux Italian Meatball Soup

This meaty goodness is super low-carb, becoming an essential soup during your winter weather blues.

## Ingredients:

- 1 spiraled zucchini
- 1 diced onion
- 30 ounces beef stock
- 3 diced celery stalks
- 1 diced tomato
- 1 diced carrot
- 2 pounds crumbled beef
- 1/3 cup shredded Parmesan cheese
- 7 minced garlic cloves
- 1 egg
- 2 tsp. onion powder
- 5 tbsp. chopped parsley
- salt and pepper to taste

## Directions:

- Begin by pouring the stock, the vegetables, and the garlic together in the slow cooker. Heat them on LOW.
- Next, form the meatballs by mixing together the egg, the salt, the onion powder, the beef, and the Parmesan. Form this mixture into meatballs.
- Next, brown the meatballs in a skillet and drop them in the slow cooker. Allow the meatballs and the rest of the soup to cook on LOW for six hours. Enjoy!

# BBQ-Based Pot Roast

This zealous BBQ pot roast brings you back down south with marvelous flavor.

**Ingredients:**

- 9 pounds beef chuck
- 1 diced onion
- 4 tbsp. butter
- 6 minced garlic cloves
- 5 tbsp. splenda
- 1 tbsp. mustard
- 3 tbsp. vinegar
- 3 tbsp. Worcestershire sauce

**Directions:**

Begin by bringing all the above ingredients together in the slow cooker and allow it to cook for ten hours on LOW. Slice the meat, and pour the sauce overtop. Enjoy!

# Super Ketogenic Vegetable and Beef Chili

This chili recipe is pulsing with delicious vegetable flavor with all the added boost of fatty and protein-revving beef!

## Ingredients:

- 1 ¾ pound ground beef
- 1 diced green pepper
- 1 diced red pepper
- 4 minced garlic cloves
- 30 ounces crushed tomatoes
- 15 ounces tomato sauce
- 15 ounces diced tomatoes
- 1 diced cup of celery
- 1 ½ minced jalapeno peppers
- 1 tbsp. basil
- 4 tbsp. chili powder
- 2 tsp. cumin
- ½ tsp. cayenne pepper

## Directions:

Bring all the above ingredients together in the slow cooker and stir well. Next, place the heat to LOW on the slow cooker and cook the chili for seven hours. Enjoy!

# Faux Cheese Beef-Based Lasagna

This lasagna has it all: vibrant vegetables, essential meat, and FAKE cheese—essential if you're lactose intolerant but still want to reap the stunning rewards of the ketogenic diet.

**Ingredients:**

**Marinara Sauce Ingredients:**

- 1/3 cup olive oil
- 2 minced garlic cloves
- 1 diced onion
- 8 cups diced tomatoes
- ¼ tbsp. honey

**Meat Ingredients:**

- ¾ pound ground beef
- 1 ½ tbsp. olive oil
- 1 diced onion
- 15 chopped basil leaves
- salt and pepper

**Faux Cheese Sauce Ingredients:**

- 1 diced onion
- 1 tbsp. olive oil
- 1 minced garlic cloves
- 1/3 cup coconut milk
- 1 egg
- 5 noodle-sliced zucchinis

**Directions:**

1. Begin by bringing the first five ingredients together in a skillet and sauté them together for about five minutes on high before reducing the heat to LOW and allowing it to cook for twenty minutes, covered.
2. Next, create the meat by sautéing the beef with the other meat ingredients. Set this to the side, as well. Next, create the cheese by forming together the last ingredients—except for the zucchini—in a sauce pan and allowing it to cook for about four minutes. Next, blend the ingredients well until you reach your cheese consistency. Next, assemble the lasagna by placing one cup of red sauce at the bottom of the slow cooker. Spread it, and then add five zucchini noodles to the very bottom. Add about a third of the cheese sauce over these noodles, and then add a third of the meat sauce. Repeat this layering process until you've used up all your lasagna. Cover the lasagna and cook it on HIGH for two hours. Serve the lasagna warm, and enjoy!

# Ketogenic Chipotle Beef

Cumin and lime juice rev in this Chipotle-restaurant-inspired beef recipe.

**Ingredients:**

- 3 pounds boneless beef chuck
- 3 tbsp. olive oil
- ½ cup water
- 1 tbsp. cumin
- 5 minced garlic cloves
- 1 tsp. oregano
- 2 tbsp. lime juice
- 1 tsp. cloves
- 4 tbsp. tomato paste

**Directions:**

First, bring all the ingredients except for the beef into a food processor. Place the beef in the food processor, and pour the created sauce overtop the beef. Place the lid on the slow cooker, and cook the beef on LOW for eight hours. Next, shred the meat, and eat it with the included sauce. Enjoy!

# Chapter 5:
# Pork Ketogenic Recipes

## Pork-Based Chili Recipe

This pork-based chili provides none of the carbohydrates of past chili days with ALL of the awesome flavor

### Ingredients:

- 9 slices bacon
- 2 ¼ pound ground pork
- 3 diced green peppers
- 1 diced onion
- 14 ounces diced tomato
- 8 ounces tomato paste
- 1 pack chili seasoning
- salt and pepper to taste

### Directions:

Begin by bringing all the above ingredients together in a slow cooker, slicing up the bacon as you go. Allow the mixture to cook for six hours on LOW, stirring every few hours. Enjoy!

# Faux Split Pea and Ham Soup

This faux split pea and ham soup is an excellent low-carb take on the once-split-pea-high-carb meal.

## Ingredients:

- 4 cups chicken broth
- 1 chicken bullion cube
- 5 cups water
- 15 ounces green beans
- 15 ounces diced cauliflower
- 2 cups diced celery
- 3 minced garlic cloves
- 3 cups diced ham
- 1 tsp. thyme
- 1 tsp. rosemary
- salt and pepper to taste

## Directions:

1. Begin by bringing the green beans, the cauliflower, the broth, the bouillon, and the water together in the slow cooker. Cook the mixture for four hours on HIGH. Next, puree this mixture in a blender.
2. Place the onion, the celery, the ham, and the garlic into the slow cooker with the blended sauce, and cook for an additional five hours on HIGH. Salt and pepper to taste, and enjoy warm.

# Apple Flavored Pork Tenderloin

Nobody said your taste buds wouldn't like the ketogenic diet. Show them a good time with apple-based pork tenderloin, and rival your best meal yet.

## Ingredients:

- 5 gala apples
- 2 pounds pork tenderloin
- 3 tbsp. honey
- 1 tsp. nutmeg

## Directions:

1. Begin by slicing the apples.
2. Place one layer of apples at the bottom of the slow cooker and add the nutmeg overtop.
3. Next, place the tenderloins over the apples. Add any additional apples overtop the tenderloin, and place the lid on the slow cooker.
4. Cook the tenderloin on LOW for eight hours. Enjoy your apple-flavored tenderloin warm.

# Mexican Style Pork Carnitas

All the flair of Mexican food comes alive in the slow cooker.

## Ingredients:

- 9 pounds pork
- 2 tbsp. cumin
- 3 tbsp. butter
- 1 diced onion
- 1 tbsp. salt
- 3 tbsp. chili powder
- 1 ½ cup water
- 4 minced garlic cloves

## Directions:

Begin by bringing all the above ingredients together into the slow cooker and cooking the pork for eight hours on HIGH. Next, tear up the meat with two forks, and enjoy.

# Classic Ketogenic Pulled Pork

This pulled pork is humming with paprika, chili powder, and low-carb BBQ for your next outdoor party.

**Ingredients:**

- 1 cup chicken broth
- 5 sliced bacon
- 2 pounds pork tenderloin
- 2 tbsp. chili powder
- 2 tbsp. paprika
- 2 cups low-carb BBQ sauce
- salt and pepper to taste

**Directions:**

Begin by pouring the broth into the slow cooker. Add the pork, and then top the pork with everything else. Place the lid on the slow cooker, and allow the pork to cook on LOW for eight hours. Shred up the pork to created "pulled" pork, and enjoy with the created sauce.

# Pork-Stuffed Green Peppers

This awesome stuffed green pepper recipe provides a new take on the traditional dish: cauliflower, instead of rice, coincides with the pork sausage beautifully.

## Ingredients:

- 1 ¼ pound ground pork sausage
- 1 can tomato paste
- 6 green peppers
- ¾ head chopped and riced cauliflower
- 4 minced garlic cloves
- 1 diced onion
- 3 tsp. diced basil
- 3 tsp. dried thyme

## Directions:

1. Begin by slicing off the "head" of each of the peppers.
2. Next, rice the cauliflower, and bring the cauliflower and the rest of the ingredients together in a large bowl. Stir well. Next, pour this mixture into the peppers, and place each of the peppers head-up in the slow cooker. Place the tops back on the peppers.
3. Next, allow the peppers to cook in the slow cooker on LOW for six hours. Enjoy!

# Pork Sausage with Collared Greens

This browned sausage and greens crockpot stew is delicious no matter the circumstances.

## Ingredients:

- ½ cup kidney beans
- 2 bunches sliced collard greens
- 1 tsp. garlic powder
- 5 pork Italian sausage links
- 1 tsp. garlic
- ½ cup water

## Directions:

Bring all the above ingredients together in a slow cooker, and cook the mixture for six hours on LOW. Next, slice up the sausage, and stir for a few moments. Cook the stew for a half hour on LOW, next, with the cover off, and enjoy.

# Super Peppered Pork Stew

This peppered pork shoulder makes an excellent stew for your next lazy day.

## Ingredients:

- 3 diced onions
- 3 ½ pounds chopped pork shoulder
- 7 minced garlic cloves
- 1 diced cabbage head
- salt and pepper
- 2 tbsp. red boat fish sauce
- 1 tbsp. balsamic vinegar
- 1/3 cup diced parsley

## Directions:

Begin by bringing all the ingredients together in the slow cooker and allowing it to cook for ten hours on LOW. Enjoy after a good stir.

# Chapter 6:
# Lamb Ketogenic Recipes

## Low-Carb Ketogenic Lamb with Tarragon

This super-spiced vegetable and lamb dish is traditional in the Middle East.

**Ingredients:**

- 2 pounds lamb
- 2 cups peeled carrot
- 1 can cannellini beans
- 1 cup diced celery
- 3 tsp. tarragon
- 3 diced garlic cloves
- salt and pepper
- 1 can diced tomatoes

**Directions:**

Begin by bringing all the ingredients together in the slow cooker on LOW for ten hours. Next, remove the juice from the slow cooker, and enjoy the lamb with the other side ingredients.

# Slow Cooked Lamb Chops

These low-carb lamb chops are pulsing with oregano, garlic, and onion flavor, leaving your taste buds and your ketogenic needs satisfied.

**Ingredients:**

- 9 lamb loin chops
- 1 diced onion
- 1 tsp. thyme
- 1 tsp. oregano
- 3 minced garlic cloves
- salt and pepper to taste

**Directions:**

Bring the above ingredients together in a slow cooker, making sure to rub the lamb chops with the appropriate spices. Cover the slow cooker and cook the lamb on LOW for four hours. Serve warm, and enjoy.

# Crock Pot Braised Lamb

Delicious braised lamb is ripe with tomato and thyme flavor.

## Ingredients:

- 1 diced onion
- 3 diced celery stalks
- 2 ½ cups chicken stock
- 4 minced garlic cloves
- 3 diced carrots
- 3 tbsp. tomato paste
- 2 bay leaves
- 3 diced tomatoes
- 5 lamb shanks
- salt and pepper to taste

## Directions:

Place the lamb in the slow cooker, and add the rest of the ingredients overtop. Allow the lamb to cook on LOW for seven hours. Next, remove the lamb, and puree all the rest of the ingredients in a blender or a food processor until smooth. Pour about half of the sauce over the lamb, and serve the rest of the sauce at the table with the lamb. Enjoy!

# Moroccan-Based Lamb Stew Recipe

Vibrant coriander and cumin rev this Moroccan-based lamb recipe to an incredible taste level.

## Ingredients:

- 3 pounds diced lamb shoulder
- 1 tbsp. cumin
- 2 tsp. salt
- 2 tsp. coriander
- 1 ½ tsp. fennel seeds
- salt and pepper
- 5 tbsp. olive oil
- 1 diced onion
- 3 cups chicken broth
- 1 ½ tbsp. tomato paste
- 5 ounces dried apricots
- 1 can chickpeas
- 3 cinnamon sticks
- 2 tsp. grated lemon peel
- ½ tbsp. ginger

## Directions:

1. Begin by coating the lamb in the first six ingredients. Next, brown the lamb in a skillet for five minutes. Place the lamb in the slow cooker, and cover it with the remaining ingredients.
2. Next, allow the lamb to cook for five hours on HIGH. Enjoy the lamb stew warm.

# Down on the Farm Lamb Stew

This vegetable-based lamb stew has a unique kick to it, taking it leaps and bounds beyond the ordinary.

**Ingredients:**

- 2 ¼ pound chopped lamb
- 1 ¼ cup diced figs
- 1 diced onion
- 3 minced garlic cloves
- 3 cups beef stock
- 1 diced cup dates
- 3 cups diced broccoli
- 1 cup diced carrots
- 2 cups diced celery
- 1 tbsp. coriander
- 2 tsp. ginger
- 1 tsp. allspice
- ¼ tsp. cayenne pepper
- salt and pepper to taste

**Directions:**

1. Begin by rubbing the lamb with all the spices. Next, place the lamb at the bottom of the slow cooker and add all the other ingredients overtop, stirring a bit as you go.
2. Place the lid on the slow cooker and allow the stew to cook on LOW for eight hours. After eight hours, stir well, and serve the stew warm. Enjoy!

# Chapter 7:
# Seafood Ketogenic Recipes

## Herbed and Poached Slow Cooked Salmon

This herbed and lemoned salmon is essential for your omega-3-rich, healthful dinner.

**Ingredients:**

- 3 cups water
- 1 diced shallot
- 1 sliced lemon
- 5 sprigs dill
- 2 ½ pounds salmon
- salt and pepper

**Directions:**

Begin by bringing all the ingredients together in the slow cooker on LOW for about one hour. Check to make sure the salmon is done and note that the salmon can remain there for another hour before removing. Enjoy warm with a bit of extra lemon overtop.

# Savory Shrimp Stew

This shrimp-based vegetable stew warms your soul with its layered flavor.

**Ingredients:**

- 3 tbsp. olive oil
- 1 pound peeled shrimp
- 3 minced garlic cloves
- 1 sliced carrot
- 1 tsp. fennel seeds
- ½ cup diced green pepper
- 1 tsp. Splenda
- 3 tbsp. diced parsley
- 1 cup water

**Directions:**

Bring the above ingredients—except for the shrimp—together in the slow cooker. Cover the slow cooker, and cook the stew on LOW for eight hours. After eight hours, add the shrimp. Cover the slow cooker and cook the stew on HIGH for thirty minutes more. Next, serve warm, and enjoy!

# Ketogenic Jambalaya

Southern Cookin' illuminates in this super ketogenic jambalaya recipe.

**Ingredients:**

- 1 diced onion
- 1 tbsp. olive oil
- 3 diced zucchinis
- 1 ½ tbsp. butter
- 7 minced garlic cloves
- 3 sliced sausages
- 3 tbsp. Cajun seasoning
- 12 cup chicken broth
- 4 diced green peppers
- 14 ounces crushed tomatoes
- ¾ pound chopped chicken breasts
- ¾ pound peeled and cooked shrimp

**Directions:**

Begin by bringing all the above ingredients together in the slow cooker, stirring well. Place the lid on the slow cooker, and allow the jambalaya to cook for eight hours on LOW before serving. Enjoy!

# Chapter 8:
# Ketogenic Dessert Recipes

Slow cooked cocoa powder and no-sugar sweetener yield a super low-carb and ketogenic dessert, perfect for your constant sweet tooth.

**Ingredients:**

- 2 cups almond flour
- 1 cup cocoa powder
- 1 cup stevia
- 2 tsp. baking powder
- 1/3 cup whey protein powder
- 4 eggs
- 1 cup almond milk
- 1/3 cup no-sugar chocolate chips
- 1 tsp. vanilla

**Directions:**

Bring all the above ingredients together in a large mixing bowl and stir well. Next, pour the batter into the slow cooker, place the lid on the slow cooker, and cook on LOW for three hours. Enjoy warm!

# Autumnal Pumpkin Pie Cake

This fall and winter-ready pumpkin pie cake is perfect for your next holiday party.

## Ingredients:

- ½ cup coconut flour
- 2 cups diced pecans
- 1 cup stevia
- 1 tsp. ginger
- 2 tsp. cinnamon
- 1/3 cup whey protein powder
- 2 tsp. baking powder
- 1 ¼ cup pumpkin puree
- 1/3 cup melted butter
- 1 tsp. vanilla
- ½ tsp. salt

## Directions:

Bring all the above ingredients together into a blender or a food processor, and blend the ingredients until they're smooth. Pour the mixture into a slow cooker and allow it to cook on LOW for three hours. Enjoy warm!

# Super Low-Carb Chocolate Fudge

This Ghirardelli melted chocolate formulates the most delicious low-carbohydrate fudge you've ever had: a must-have for all holiday treats.

**Ingredients:**

- 5 tbsp. salted butter
- 3 squares unsweetened Ghirardelli chocolate
- 4 scoops chocolate protein powder
- 1 ½ tsp. stevia
- 7 ounces Neufchatel cheese

**Directions:**

1. Begin by melting the butter in a saucepan. Next, bring all the ingredients together in a slow cooker, stir well, and place the lid on the slow cooker. Allow the mixture to cook on LOW for one hour.
2. Next, Remove the mixture, and then fill a baking dish with the fudge. Place the baking dish in the freezer, and allow it to harden before serving. Enjoy!

# Conclusion

These 50 Slow Cooker Ketogenic Diet Recipes will take your body on a journey to refined weight loss. As your ketone levels elevate in your blood stream, your body will have an easy time stripping you of the weight you've gained as a result of our preservative-laden and super-high-carbohydrate society. Understand the benefits moving forward and further remember: none of these slow cooker recipes take more than about ten minutes to put together. Just toss all the awesome, healthful ingredients into your slow cooker, head out for the day, and come back to a delicious meal. Measure your ketones as you go, remember to stay away from high-carbohydrate meals, and continue to fight the good fight. Weight loss comes readily on the ketogenic diet. Are you ready for it?

## My Thanks To You

I would like to thank you for buying my book. I hope you have gained a lot of value from it. If you enjoyed this book, I would like to ask you a favor. Would you be kind enough to leave a review for it? It would be greatly appreciated!

How you can leave a review:

https://www.amazon.com/gp/css/order-history and click on digital orders

Just click the link above and it will take you straight to your amazon account.

Reviews are so important to authors like myself and it would mean the world to me if you could share your feedback.

Lots of love,
**Jenn Smith**

Made in the USA
Lexington, KY
14 May 2017